Noella Faye

Copyright protected. All rights reserved. Electronic or printed reproduction is prohibited without written consent from the author.

Join us at:
https://www.subscribepage.com/noellafayecoloring
For a Free Motivational Words Mini-Pack of Printable Coloring Designs
Plus More Goodies!

THIS FUNNY NURSE SAYINGS COLORING BOOK BELONGS TO:

_____

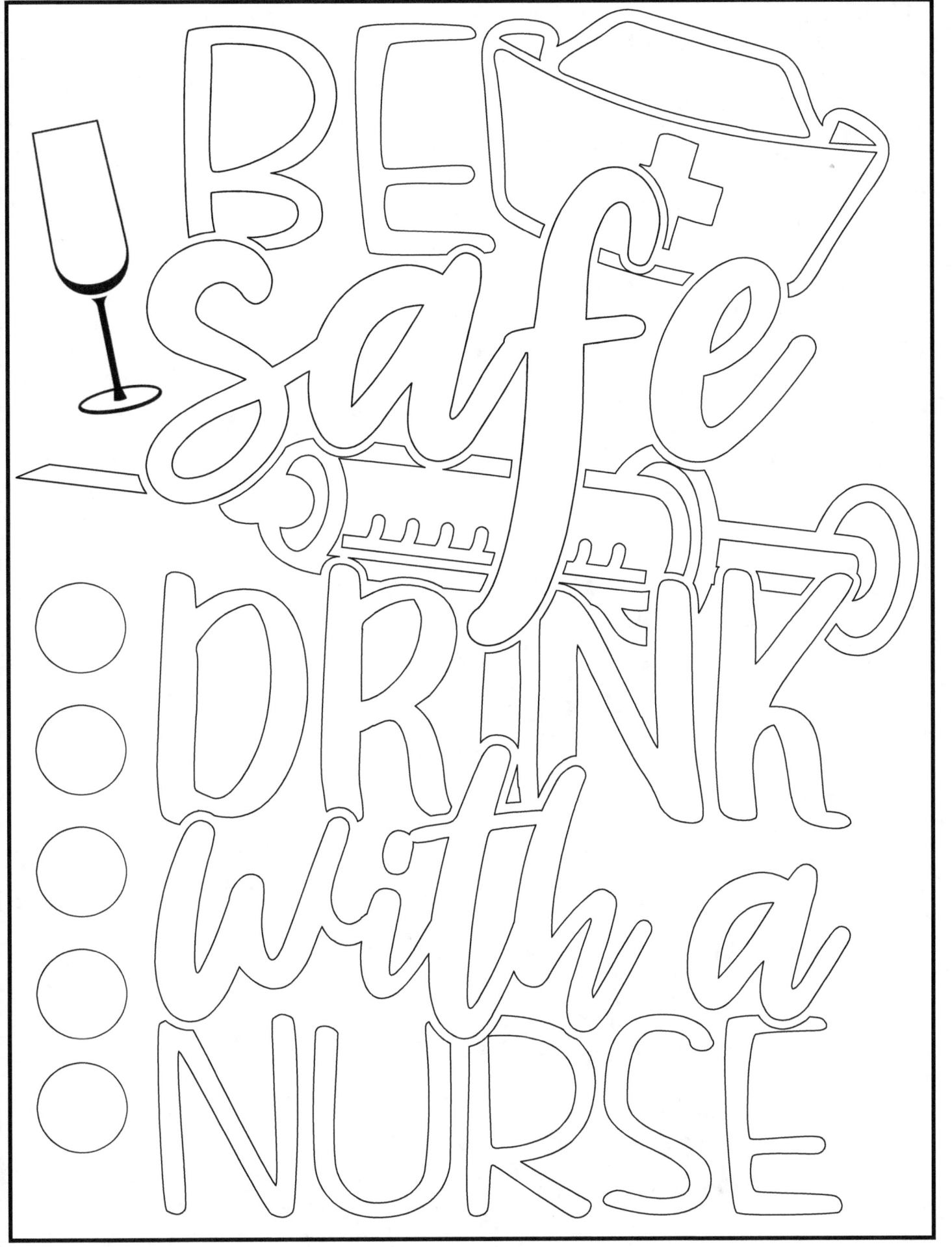

Nurse Hair Don't Care

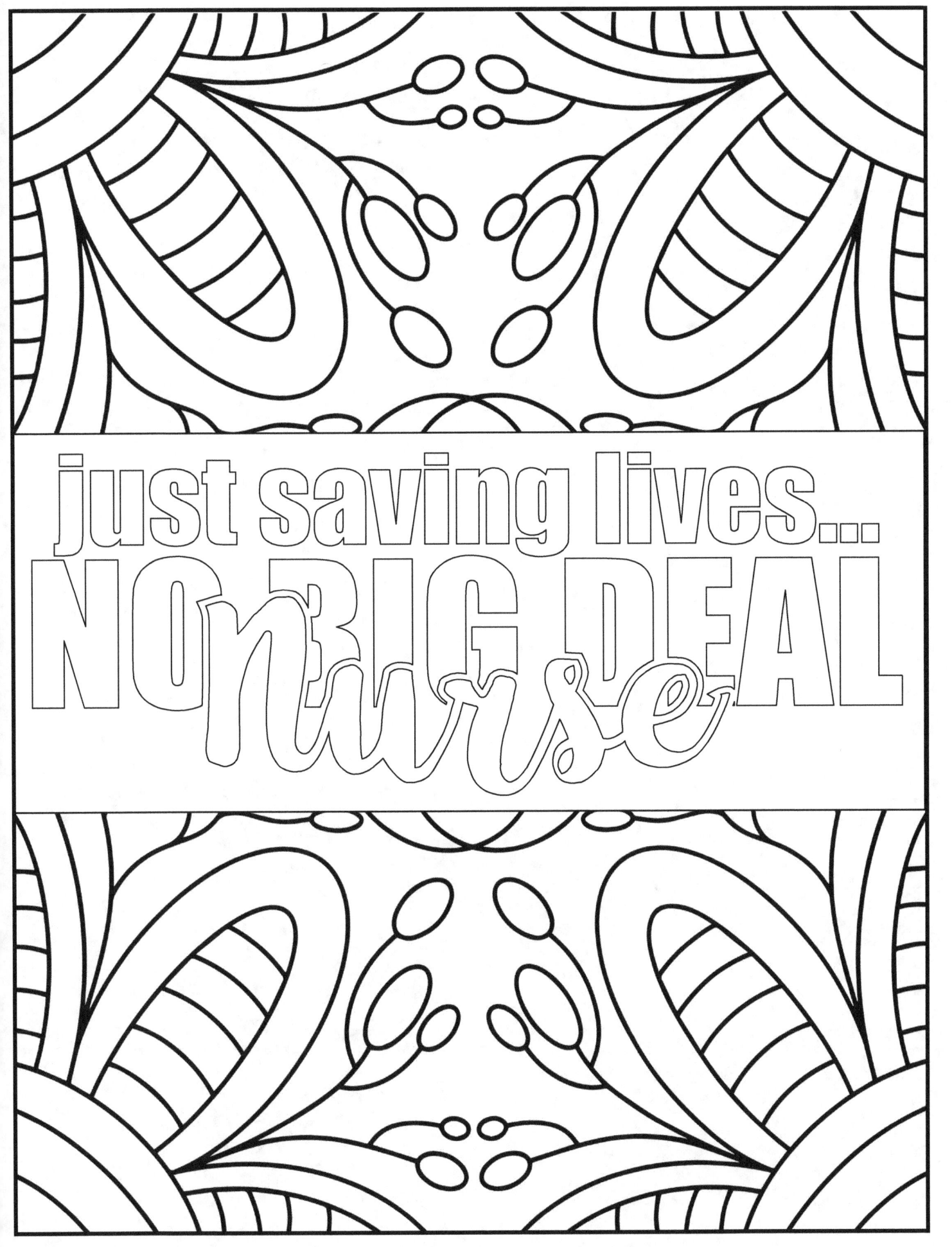

I stab people for a living

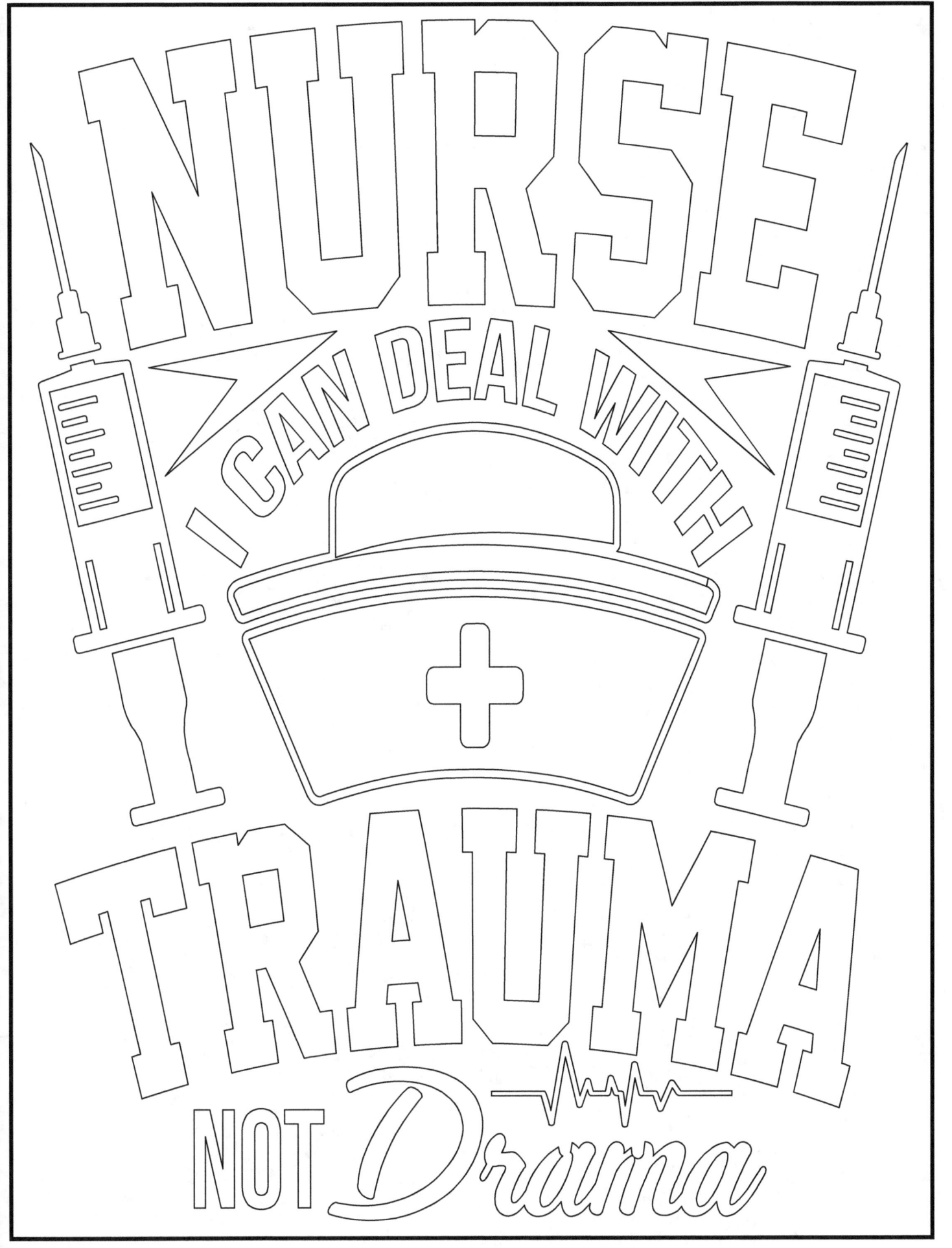

DON'T FLATTER Yourself I WAS LOOKING AT YOUR VEINS

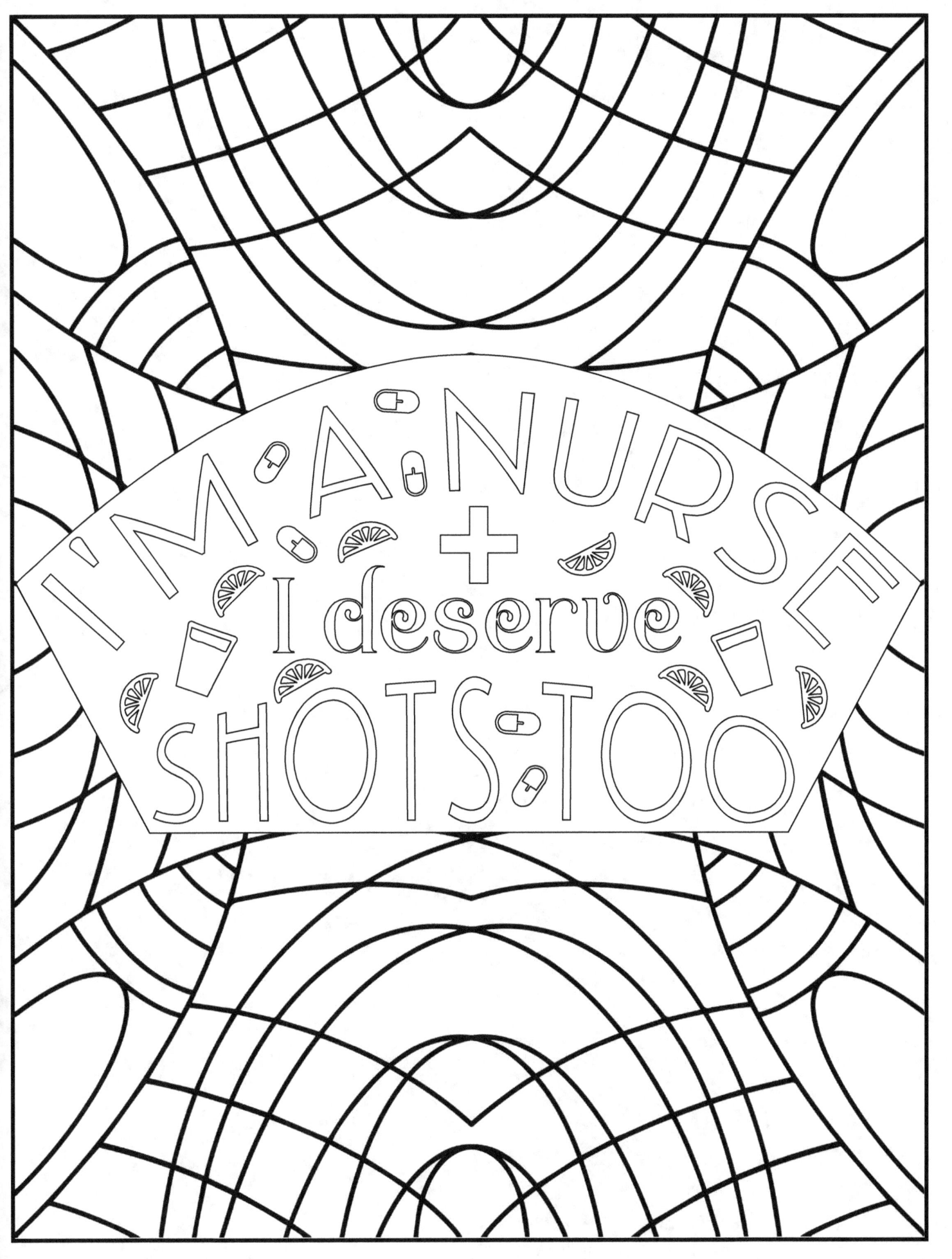

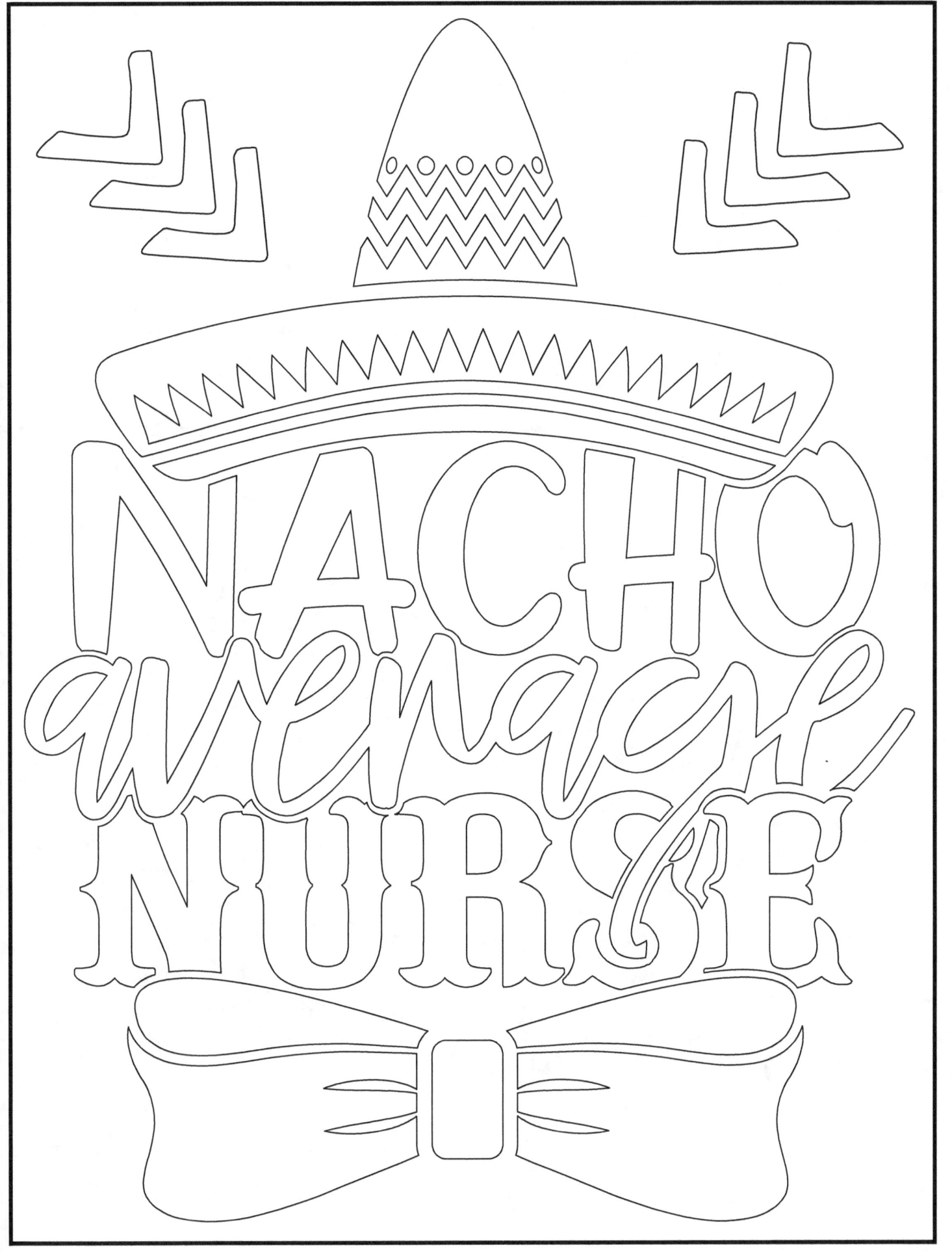

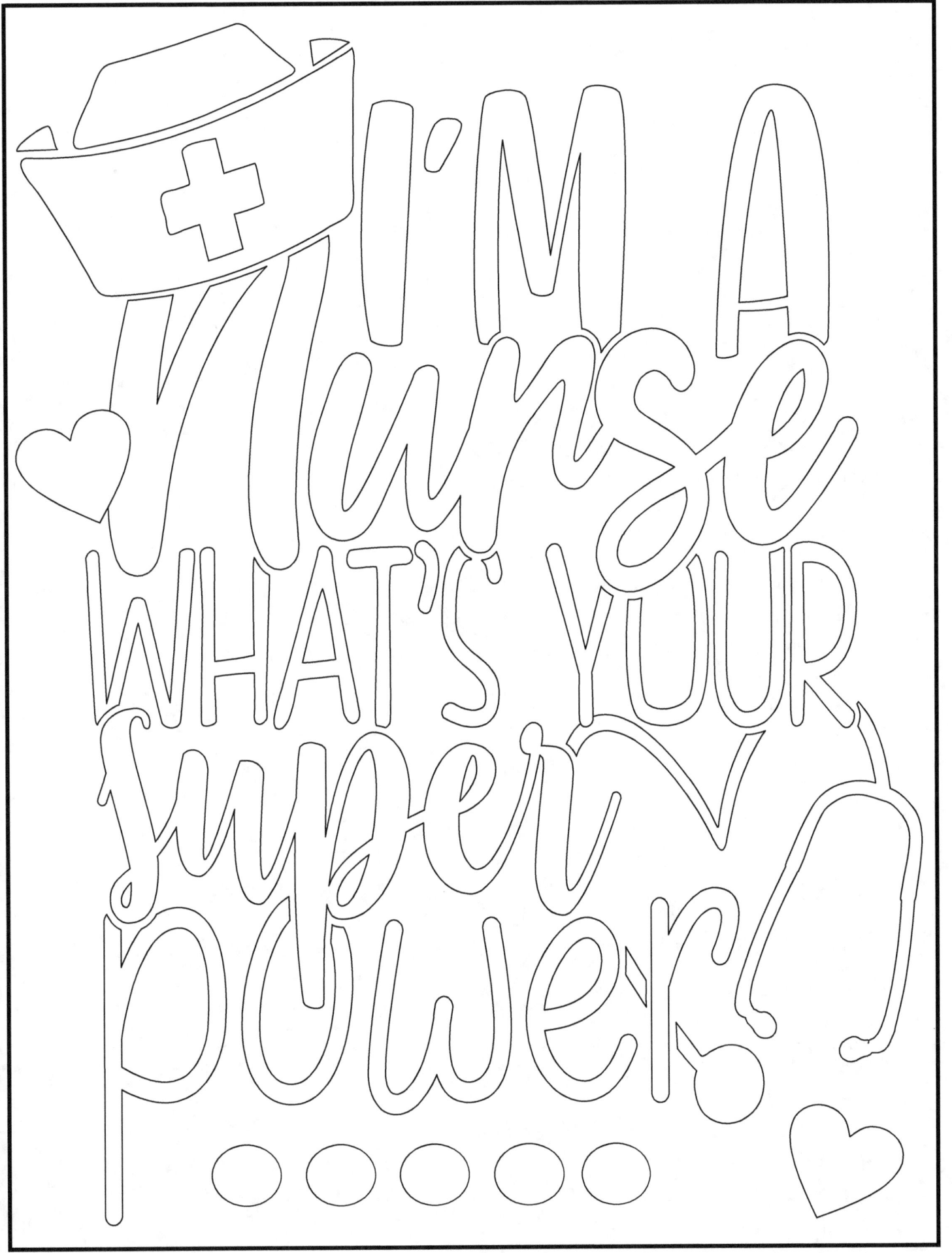

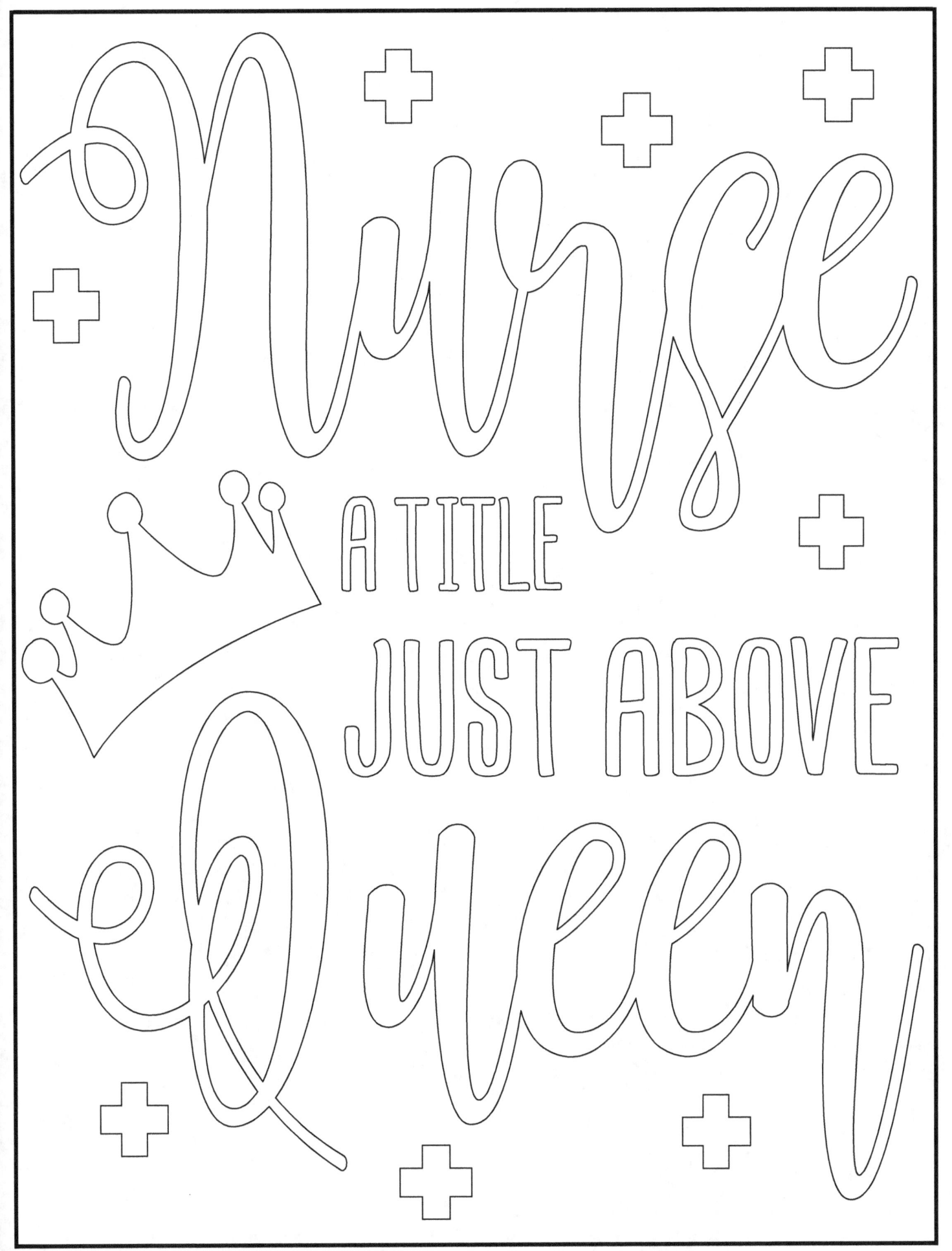

SORRY The Nice Nurse Is On Vacation

NURSE
fixin' cuts AND *stickin'* BUTTS

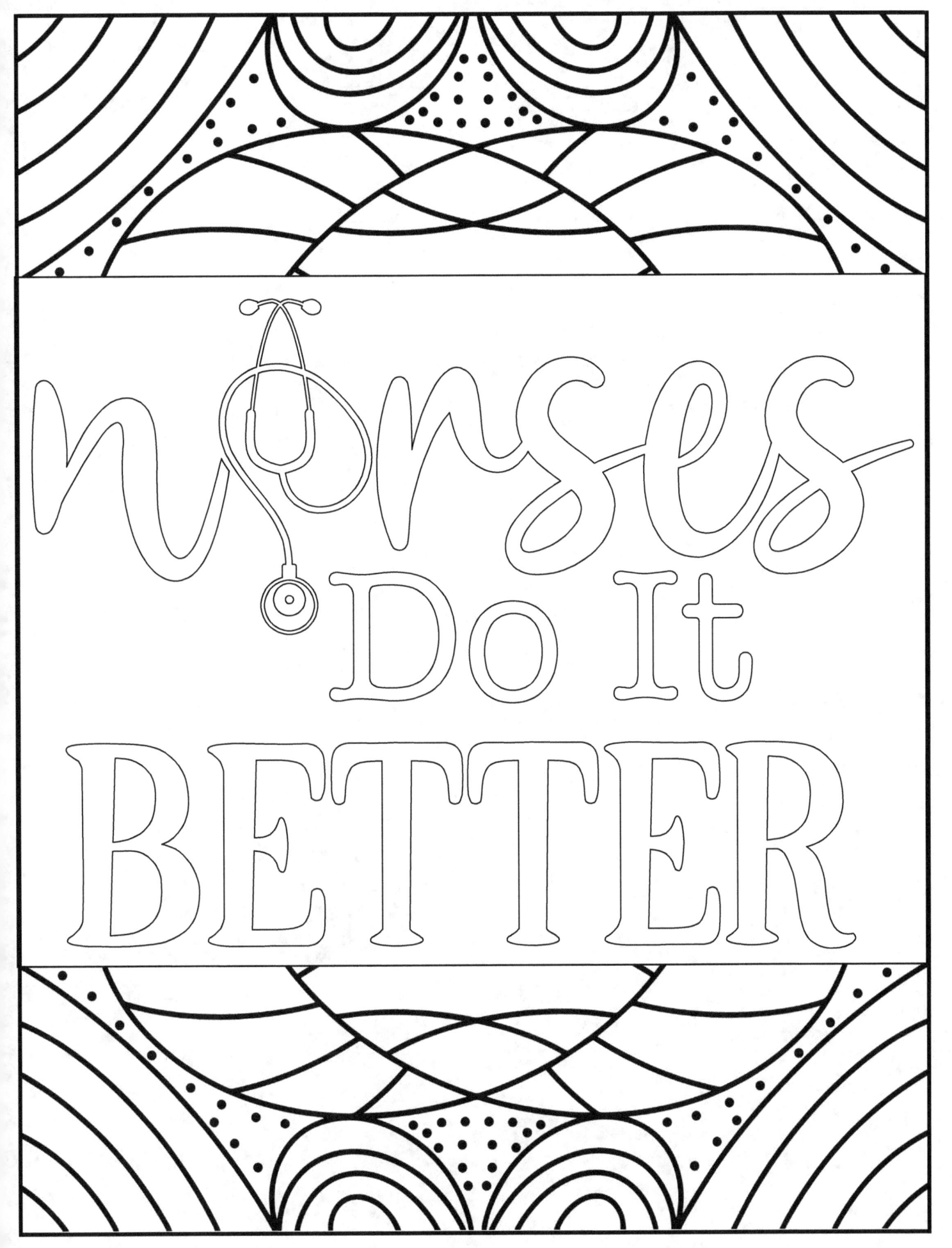

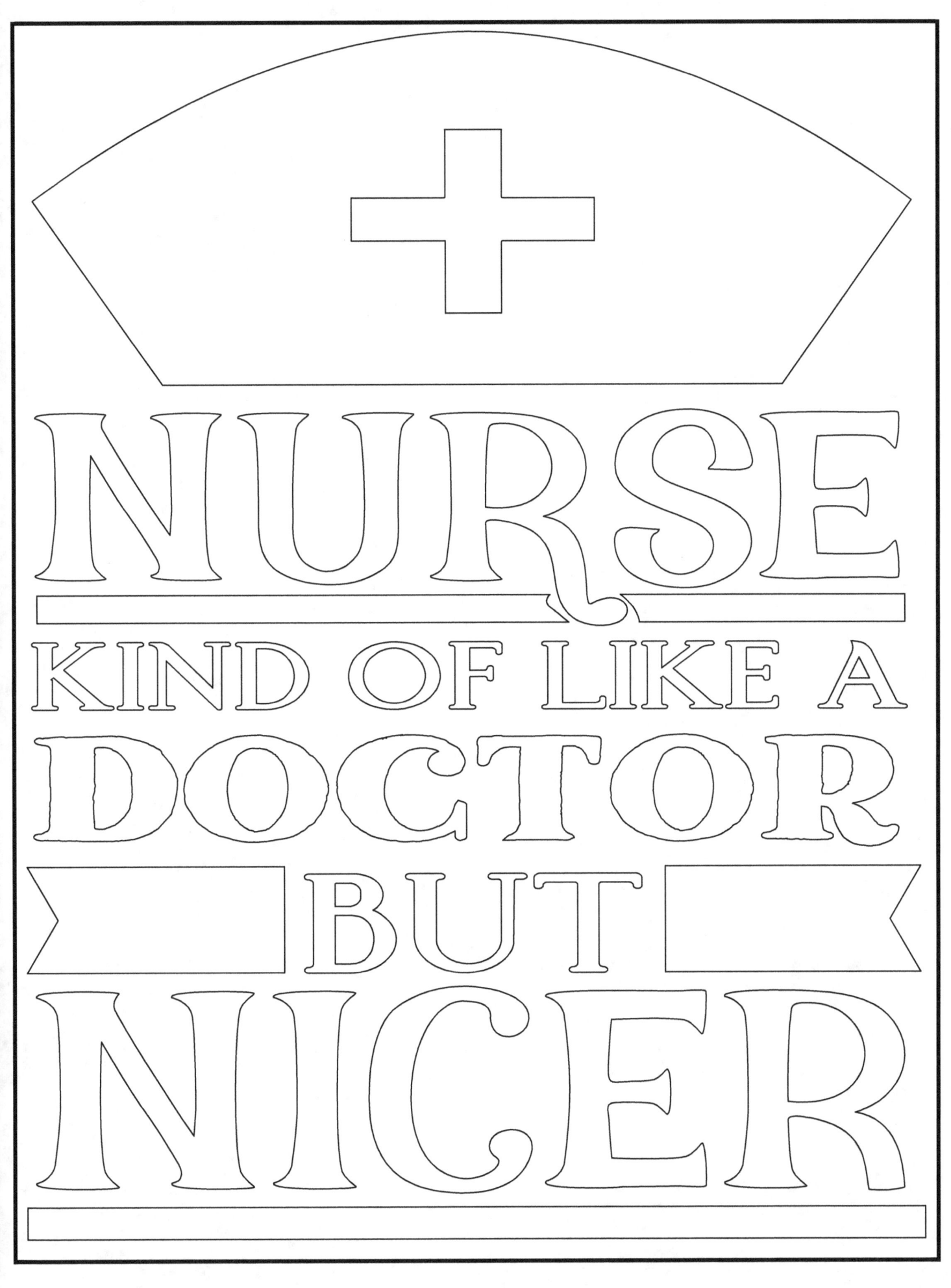

YEAH I'M THAT NURSE SORRY NOT SORRY

WILL TRADE MEDICAL ADVICE FOR WINE

NURSES

WE CAN'T FIX

Stupid

BUT WE CAN SEDATE IT

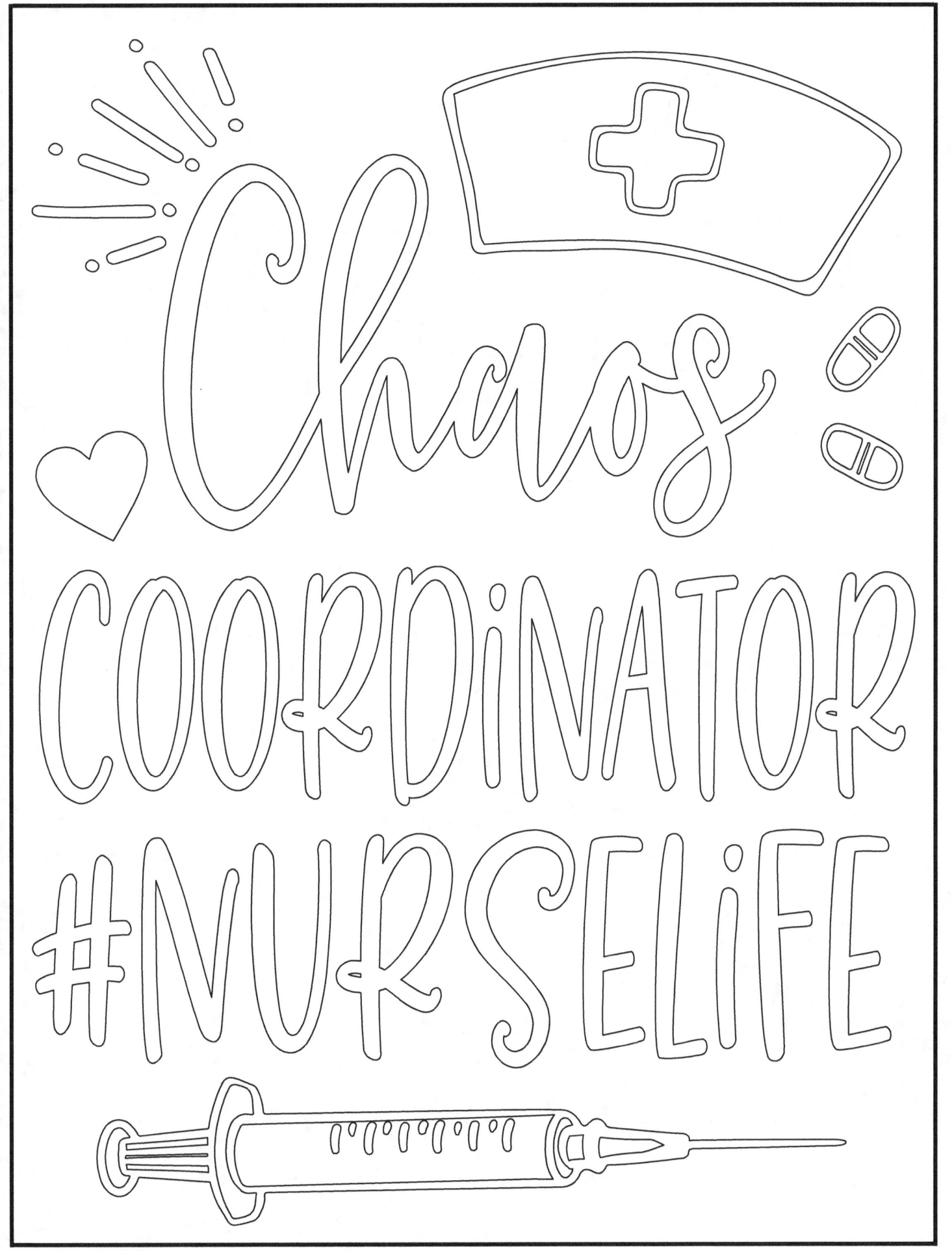

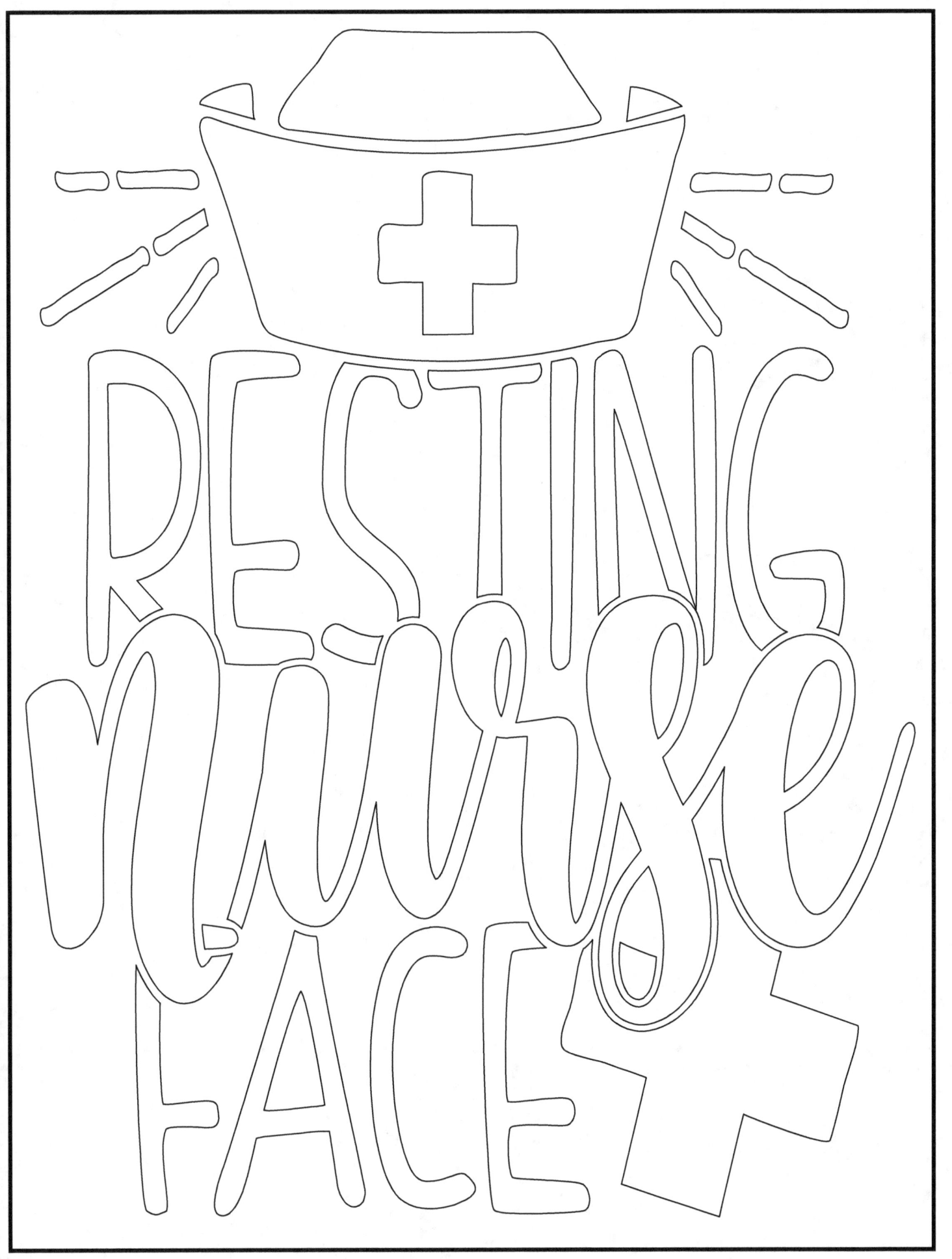

50% NURSE 50% coffee

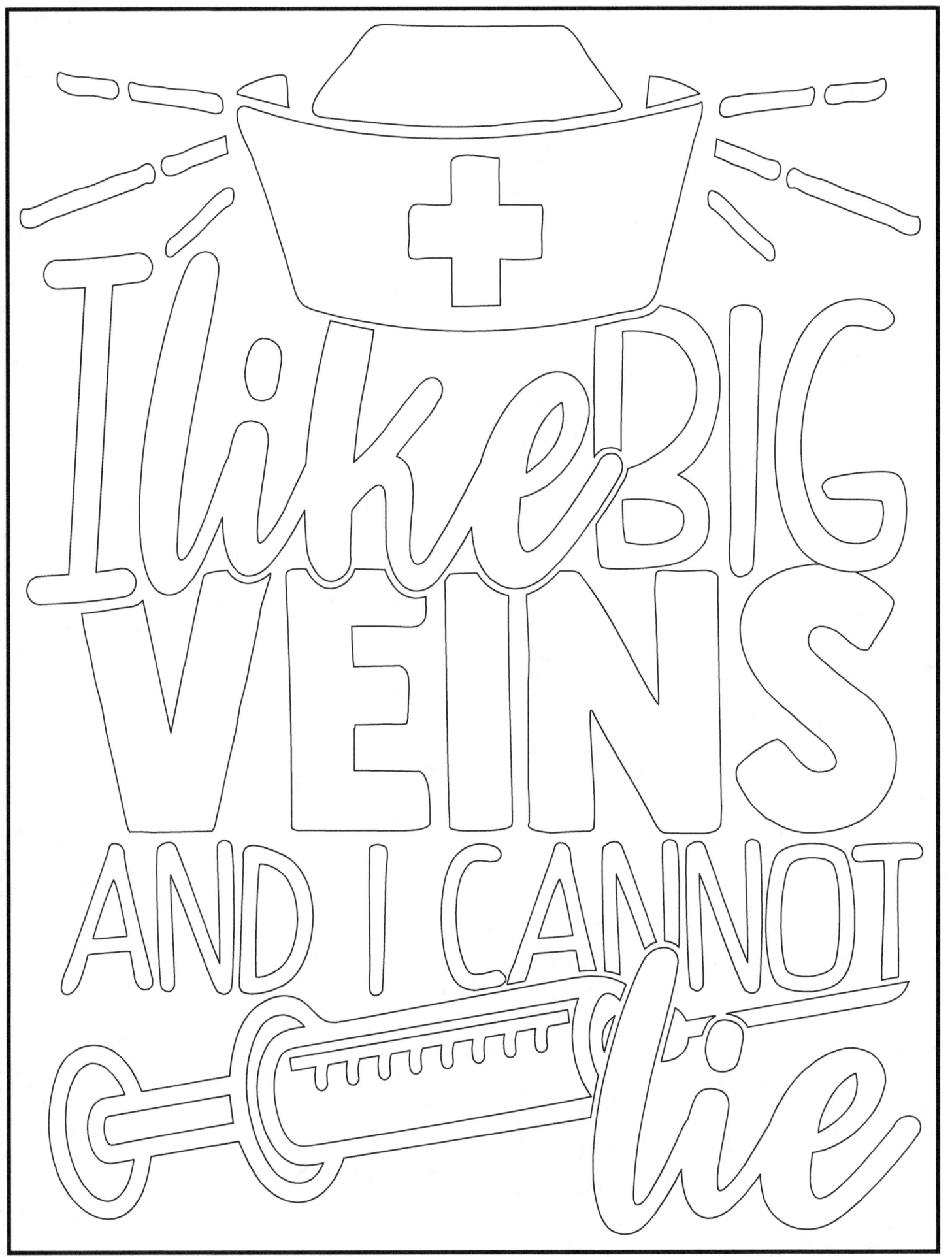

I BECAME A NURSE FOR THE FORTUNE AND FAME

Nurse because SUPERHERO isn't an OFFICIAL JOB TITLE

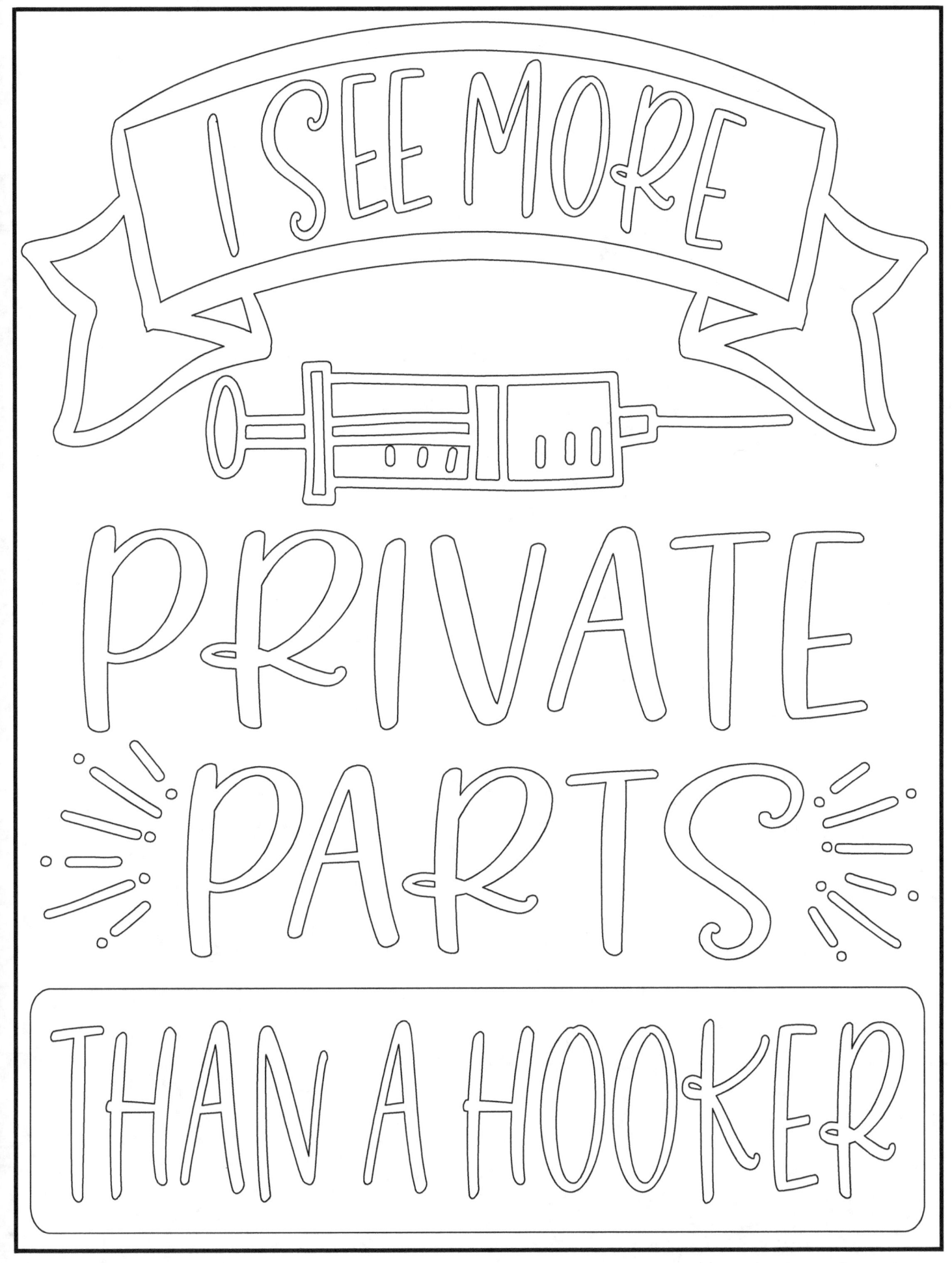

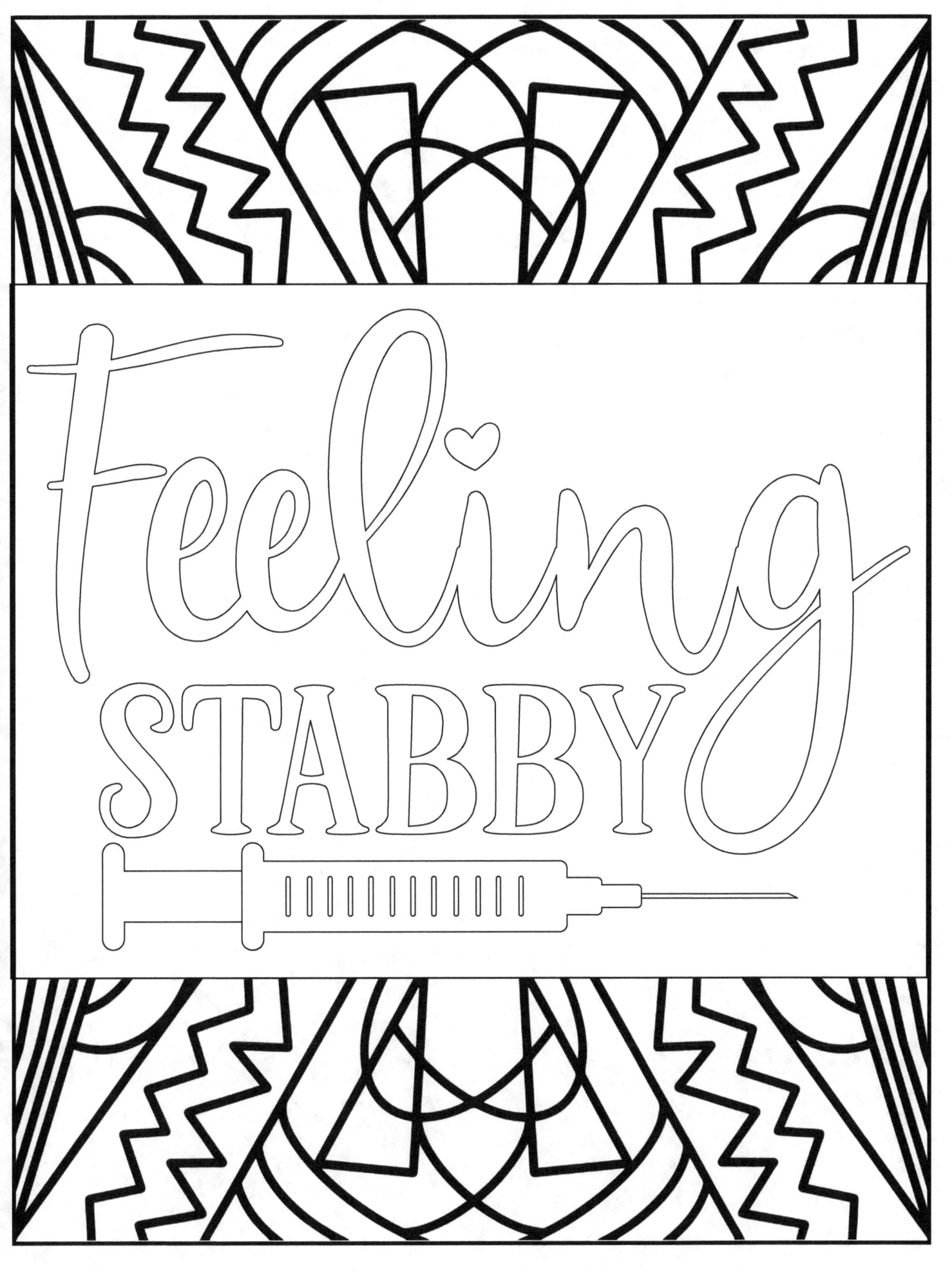

My Blood Type is Coffee

Cute enough to stop your heart, skilled enough to restart it

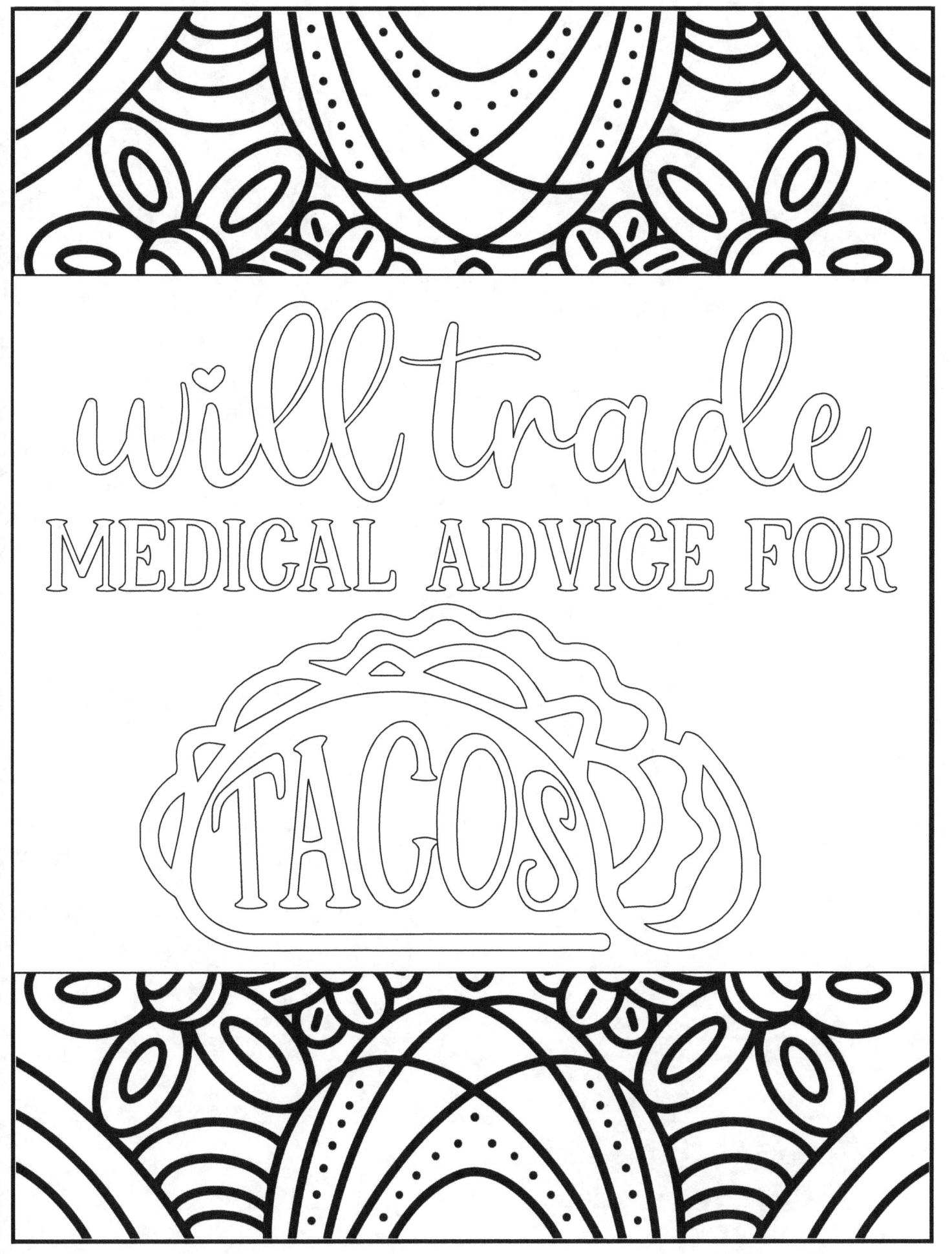

Nurses are like Pineapples

Tough on the outside, Sweet on the inside

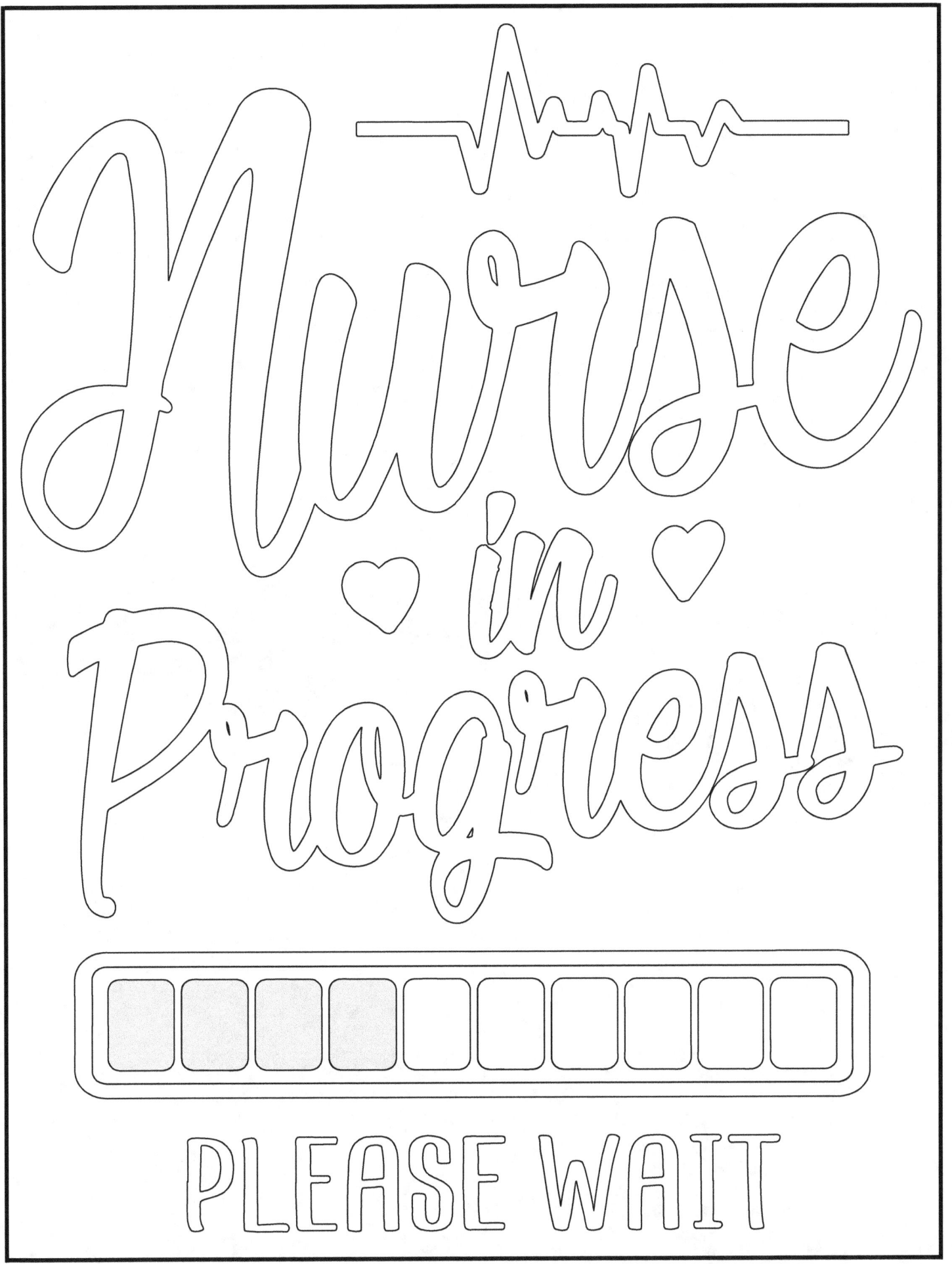

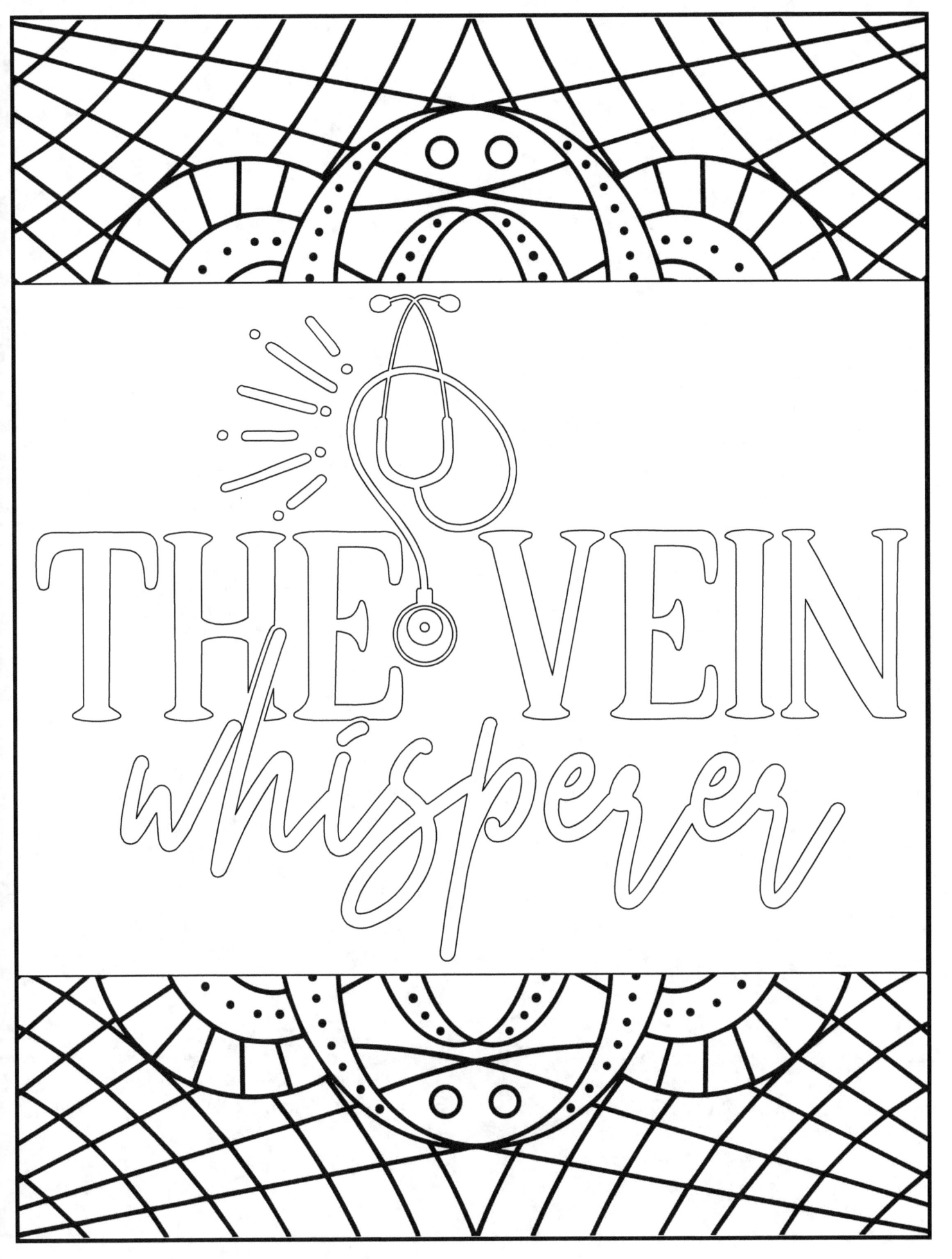

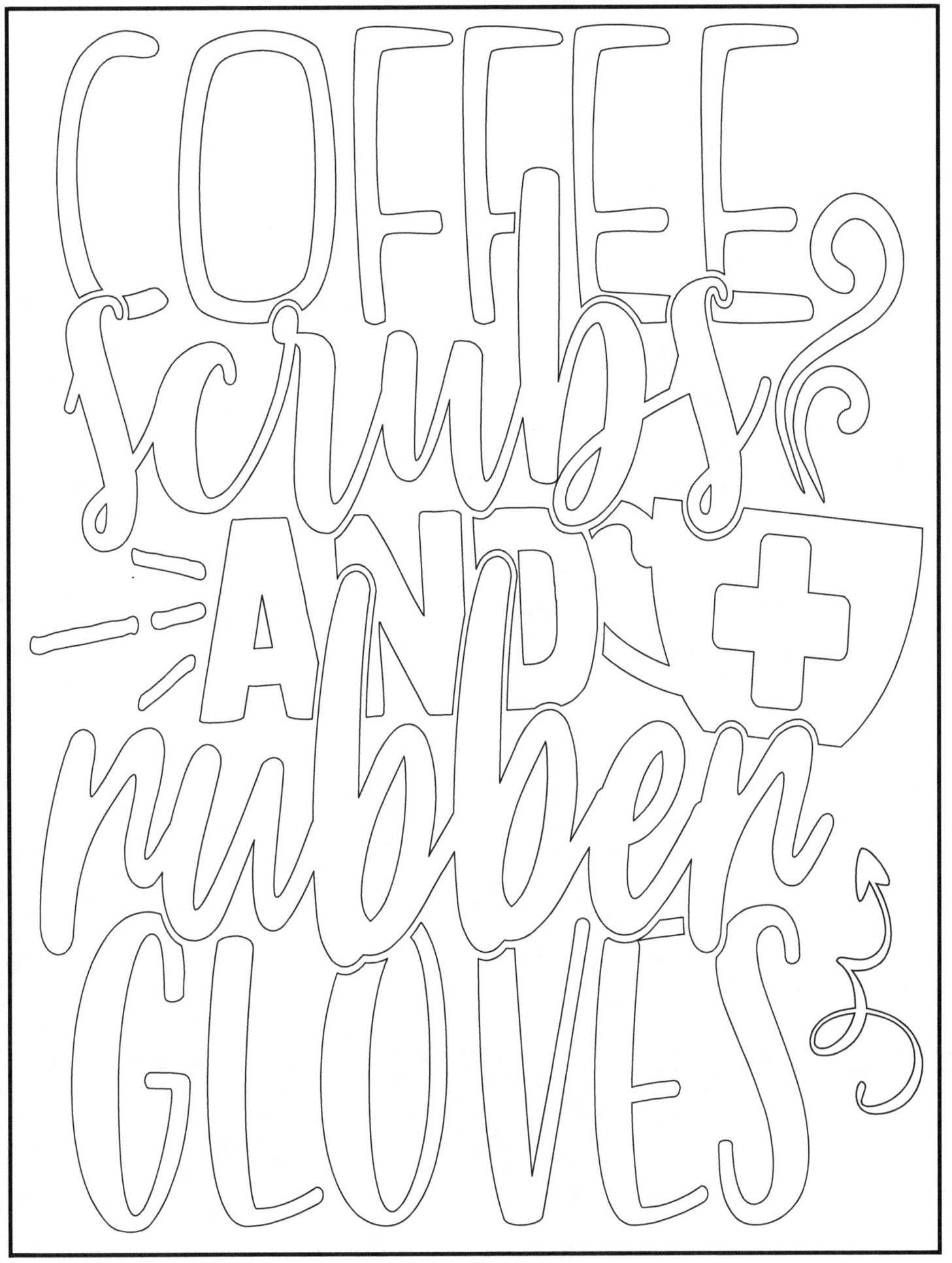

Educated Drug Dealer Nurse

Don't mess with me I get paid to stab people

SKILLED ENOUGH TO BECOME A *nurse* CRAZY ENOUGH TO *love* IT

www.ingramcontent.com/pod-product-compliance
Lightning Source LLC
Chambersburg PA
CBHW080522220526
45465CB00006B/2568